JUICING AND SMOOTHIES FOR ASTHMA

Healthy and delicious fruit blends to alleviate breathing problems and manage respiratory symptoms

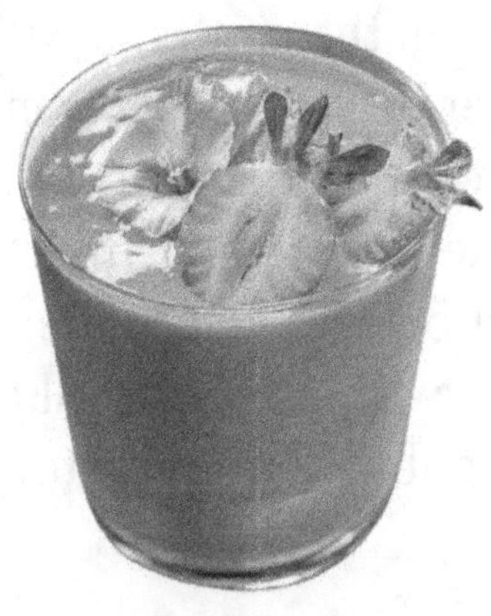

Dr. Malvin Harison

TABLE OF CONTENT

Chapter 2: 30 mouthwatering Smoothie Recipes for asthma **32**

Introduction

Welcome to "Asthma Juicing and Smoothies for Beginners," a guide that invites you to explore the transformative power of nature's elixirs on the journey to better respiratory health. In the symphony of fruits, vegetables, and superfoods, we've curated a collection of recipes specifically designed to breathe new life into your wellness routine.

Managing asthma goes beyond inhalers and prescriptions; it's about nourishing your body with the right blend of ingredients that support respiratory function. In these pages, we'll embark on a flavorful expedition, discovering how the vibrant hues of fruits and greens can become a vital part of your asthma management strategy.

Whether you're new to juicing or a blending enthusiast, our carefully crafted recipes cater to all levels of expertise. Let's turn the page to a world where each sip is a breath of fresh air, a step towards embracing the synergy of taste and health. Get ready to blend, sip, and breathe your way to a healthier, more vibrant life. The journey begins now.

The importance of taking the right juicing and smoothie

The importance of choosing the right juicing and smoothie recipes for beginners managing asthma cannot be overstated. In this holistic approach to respiratory wellness, the selection of ingredients is more than just a matter of taste – it's a strategic decision to support and enhance your respiratory health.

The carefully curated recipes in this book aim to harness the power of nature's remedies. By incorporating fruits, vegetables, and superfoods known for their anti-inflammatory and antioxidant properties, you are providing your body with the tools it needs to fortify lung function and ease the challenges of asthma.

Beyond the refreshing flavors, the simplicity and accessibility of juicing and smoothies make them an ideal addition to the daily routine of asthma management. These recipes offer a delicious and convenient way to supplement traditional treatments, promoting overall well-being and contributing to a proactive approach in maintaining respiratory health.

Chapter 1:30 delicious Asthma Juicing Recipes

Juicing can be a wonderful way to incorporate nutrient-rich ingredients into your diet that may help alleviate symptoms of asthma. Here are 30 juicing recipes that are easy to make, packed with flavor, and beneficial for respiratory health;

1. Green Goddess Juice

Ingredients:
- 2 cups spinach
- 1 cucumber
- 2 green apples
- 1 lemon (juiced)
- 1-inch piece of ginger

Instructions:
1. Wash all the ingredients thoroughly.
2. Cut the cucumber and green apples into smaller pieces.
3. Add all the ingredients to your juicer.
4. Stir well and serve immediately.

Serving: 1 glass
Nutritional Value: High in vitamins A and C, and antioxidants.
Preparation Time: 5 minutes

2. Carrot-Orange Delight

Ingredients:
- 4 carrots
- 2 oranges (peeled)
- 1-inch piece of turmeric root
Instructions:
1. Wash and peel the carrots and oranges.
2. Cut them into smaller pieces.
3. Add all the ingredients to your juicer.
4. Stir well and serve chilled.
Serving: 1 glass
Nutritional Value: Rich in beta-carotene, vitamin C, and anti-inflammatory properties.
Preparation Time: 5 minutes

3. Pineapple-Basil Blast

Ingredients:
- 2 cups pineapple chunks
- 1 handful of fresh basil leaves
- 1 lime (juiced)

Instructions:
1. Cut the pineapple into chunks.
2. Wash the basil leaves.
3. Add the pineapple chunks and basil leaves to your juicer.
4. Squeeze the lime juice into the mixture.
5. Stir well and serve over ice.

Serving: 1 glass
Nutritional Value: High in bromelain, vitamin C, and anti-inflammatory properties.
Preparation Time: 5 minutes

4. Berry-Licious juice

Ingredients:
- 1 cup of different berries (strawberries, blueberries, raspberries)
- 1 banana

- 1 cup almond milk

Instructions:

1. Wash the berries.

2. Peel and slice the banana.

3. Add the berries, banana, and almond milk to a blender.

4. Blend until smooth.

5. Serve chilled.

Serving: 1 glass

Nutritional Value: High in antioxidants, vitamins, and fiber.

Preparation Time: 5 minutes

5. Ginger-Turmeric Elixir

Ingredients:

- 1-inch piece of ginger
- 1-inch piece of turmeric root
- 2 lemons (juiced)
- 1 tablespoon honey (optional)

Instructions:

1. Peel the ginger and turmeric root.

2. Cut them into smaller pieces.

3. Add the ginger, turmeric, and lemon juice to your juicer.

4. Stir in honey, if desired.

5. Stir well and serve chilled.

Serving: 1 glass

Nutritional Value: Anti-inflammatory, immune-boosting, and antioxidant properties.

Preparation Time: 5 minutes

6. Spinach-Apple Refresher

Ingredients:
- 2 cups spinach
- 2 green apples
- 1 cucumber
- 1 lemon (juiced)

Instructions:
1. Wash all the ingredients thoroughly.
2. Cut the green apples and cucumber into smaller pieces.
3. Add all the ingredients to your juicer.
4. Stir well and serve over ice.

Serving: 1 glass

Nutritional Value: High in vitamins A, C, and K, and iron.

Preparation Time: 5 minutes

7. Beet-Berry Booster

Ingredients:
- 1 beet (peeled and chopped)
- 1 cup mixed berries (strawberries, blueberries, raspberries)
- 1 orange (peeled)
- 1 tablespoon chia seeds

Instructions:
1. Wash the beet and berries.
2. Peel and slice the orange.
3. Add the beet, berries, orange, and chia seeds to your juicer.
4. Stir well and serve chilled.

Serving: 1 glass
Nutritional Value: High in antioxidants, fiber, and essential nutrients.
Preparation Time: 5 minutes

8. Minty Watermelon Cooler

Ingredients:
- 2 cups watermelon chunks
- 1 handful of fresh mint leaves
- 1 lime (juiced)

Instructions:

1. Cut the watermelon into chunks.

2. Wash the mint leaves.

3. Add the watermelon chunks and mint leaves to your juicer.

4. Squeeze the lime juice into the mixture.

5. Stir well and serve over ice.

Serving: 1 glass

Nutritional Value: Hydrating, rich in vitamins A and C, and refreshing.

Preparation Time: 5 minutes

9. Green Goddess Detox

Ingredients:

- 2 cups spinach

- 1 cucumber

- 2 green apples

- 1 lemon (juiced)

- 1-inch piece of ginger

- Handful of fresh mint leaves

Instructions:

1. Wash the spinach, cucumber, apples, and mint leaves.

2. Cut the cucumber and apples into smaller pieces.

3. Add the spinach, cucumber, apples, lemon juice, ginger, and mint leaves to your juicer.

4. Stir well and serve over ice.

Serving: 1 glass

Nutritional Value: Detoxifying, high in antioxidants, and aids digestion.

Preparation Time: 5 minutes

10. Citrus-Berry Blast

Ingredients:

- 2 oranges (peeled)
- 1 cup mixed berries (strawberries, blueberries, raspberries)
- 1 tablespoon flax seeds

Instructions:

1. Peel the oranges and wash the berries.

2. Add the oranges, berries, and flaxseeds to your juicer.

3. Stir well and serve chilled.

Serving: 1 glass

Nutritional Value: High in vitamin C, antioxidants, and omega-3 fatty acids.

Preparation Time: 5 minutes

11. Cucumber-Mint Refresher

Ingredients:
- 1 cucumber
- 1 green apple
- 1 handful of fresh mint leaves
- 1 lime (juiced)

Instructions:
1. Wash the cucumber and mint leaves.
2. Cut the cucumber and green apple into smaller pieces.
3. Add the cucumber, green apple, mint leaves, and lime juice to your juicer.
4. Stir well and serve over ice.

Serving: 1 glass
Nutritional Value: Hydrating, refreshing, and rich in vitamins A and C.
Preparation Time: 5 minutes

12. Papaya-Ginger Zinger

Ingredients:
- 1 cup papaya chunks
- 1-inch piece of ginger

- 1 lemon (juiced)
- 1 tablespoon honey (optional)

Instructions:

1. Cut the papaya into chunks.
2. Peel and slice the ginger.
3. Add the papaya, ginger, lemon juice, and honey (if desired) to your juicer.
4. Stir well and serve chilled.

Serving: 1 glass

Nutritional Value: Anti-inflammatory, aids digestion, and boosts immune function.

Preparation Time: 5 minutes

13. Spinach-Pineapple Paradise

Ingredients:

- 2 cups spinach
- 2 cups pineapple chunks
- 1 green apple
- 1 lemon (juiced)

Instructions:

1. Wash the spinach and cut the pineapple and green apple into smaller pieces.

2. Add the spinach, pineapple chunks, green apple, and lemon juice to your juicer.

3. Stir well and serve over ice.

Serving: 1 glass

Nutritional Value: High in vitamins A, C, and B6, and aids digestion.

Preparation Time: 5 minutes

14. Carrot-Ginger Elixir

Ingredients:

- 4 carrots
- 1-inch piece of ginger
- 1 orange (peeled)
- 1 tablespoon turmeric powder

Instructions:

1. Wash and peel the carrots and orange.

2. Slice the ginger.

3. Add the carrots, ginger, orange, and turmeric powder to your juicer.

4. Stir well and serve chilled.

Serving: 1 glass

Nutritional Value: Anti-inflammatory, aids digestion, and boosts immune function.

Preparation Time: 5 minutes

15. Blueberry-Kale Powerhouse

Ingredients:
- 1 cup blueberries
- 2 cups kale leaves
- 1 banana
- 1 cup almond milk

Instructions:
1. Wash the blueberries and kale leaves.
2. Peel and slice the banana.
3. Add the blueberries, kale leaves, banana, and almond milk to a blender.
4. Blend until smooth.
5. Serve chilled.

Serving: 1 glass

Nutritional Value: High in antioxidants, vitamins, and fiber.

Preparation Time: 5 minutes

16. Mango-Coconut Dream

Ingredients:
- 1 ripe mango
- 1 cup coconut water

- 1 tablespoon lime juice
- 1 teaspoon honey (optional)

Instructions:

1. Peel and chop the mango.

2. Add the mango, coconut water, lime juice, and honey (if desired) to a blender.

3. Blend until smooth.

4. Serve chilled.

Serving: 1 glass

Nutritional Value: Rich in vitamin C, fiber, and electrolytes.

Preparation Time: 5 minutes

17. Apple-Carrot-Ginger Refresher

Ingredients:

- 2 green apples
- 2 carrots
- 1-inch piece of ginger
- 1 tablespoon lemon juice

Instructions:

1. Wash the apples, carrots, and ginger.

2. Cut the apples and carrots into smaller pieces.

3. Add the apples, carrots, ginger, and lemon juice to your juicer.

4. Stir well and serve over ice.

Serving: 1 glass

Nutritional Value: High in antioxidants, vitamins A and C, and aids digestion.

Preparation Time: 5 minutes

18. Strawberry-Basil Bliss

Ingredients:
- 1 cup strawberries
- 1 handful of fresh basil leaves
- 1 orange (peeled)
- 1 tablespoon honey (optional)

Instructions:

1. Wash the strawberries and basil leaves.

2. Peel the orange.

3. Add the strawberries, basil leaves, orange, and honey (if desired) to your juicer.

4. Stir well and serve chilled.

Serving: 1 glass

Nutritional Value: Rich in antioxidants, vitamin C, and anti-inflammatory properties.
Preparation Time: 5 minutes

19. Watermelon-Cucumber Cooler

Ingredients:
- 2 cups watermelon chunks
- 1 cucumber
- 1 lime (juiced)
- Fresh mint leaves for garnish

Instructions:
1. Cut the watermelon into chunks.
2. Wash and slice the cucumber.
3. Add the watermelon chunks, cucumber, and lime juice to your juicer.
4. Stir well and serve over ice.
5. Garnish with fresh mint leaves.
Serving: 1 glass
Nutritional Value: Hydrating, refreshing, and rich in vitamins A and C.
Preparation Time: 5 minutes

20. Pineapple-Carrot-Orange Burst

Ingredients:
- 2 cups pineapple chunks
- 2 carrots
- 2 oranges (peeled)
- 1 tablespoon turmeric powder

Instructions:
1. Wash and cut the pineapple into chunks.
2. Peel and chop the carrots and oranges.
3. Add the pineapple chunks, carrots, oranges, and turmeric powder to your juicer.
4. Stir well and serve chilled.

Serving: 1 glass

Nutritional Value: High in vitamin C, beta-carotene, and anti-inflammatory properties.

Preparation Time: 5 minutes

21. Kale-Mint Detoxifier

Ingredients:
- 2 cups kale leaves
- 1 green apple
- 1 cucumber
- 1 tablespoon lemon juice
- Handful of fresh mint leaves

Instructions:
1. Wash the kale leaves and mint leaves.
2. Cut the green apple and cucumber into smaller pieces.
3. Add the kale leaves, green apple, cucumber, lemon juice, and mint leaves to your juicer.
4. Stir well and serve over ice.

Serving: 1 glass

Nutritional Value: Detoxifying, rich in vitamins A and C, and aids digestion.

Preparation Time: 5 minutes

22. Peach-Raspberry Refresher

Ingredients:
- 2 ripe peaches
- 1 cup raspberries

- 1 tablespoon lime juice
- 1 teaspoon honey (optional)

Instructions:

1. Wash the peaches and raspberries.
2. Remove the pits from the peaches and chop them.
3. Add the peaches, raspberries, lime juice, and honey (if desired) to a blender.
4. Blend until smooth.
5. Serve chilled.

Serving: 1 glass

Nutritional Value: High in antioxidants, vitamin C, and fiber.

Preparation Time: 5 minutes

23. Spinach-Berry Blast

Ingredients:

- 2 cups spinach
- 1 cup mixed berries (strawberries, blueberries, raspberries)
- 1 banana
- 1 cup almond milk

Instructions:

1. Wash the spinach and berries.

2. Peel and slice the banana.
3. Add the spinach, berries, banana, and almond milk to a blender.
4. Blend until smooth.
5. Serve chilled.
Serving: 1 glass
Nutritional Value: High in antioxidants, vitamins, and fiber.
Preparation Time: 5 minutes

24. Turmeric-Orange Elixir

Ingredients:
- 2 oranges (peeled)
- 1-inch piece of turmeric root
- 1 lemon (juiced)
- 1 tablespoon honey (optional)

Instructions:
1. Peel the oranges and lemon.
2. Slice the turmeric root.
3. Add the oranges, turmeric root, lemon juice, and honey (if desired) to your juicer.
4. Stir well and serve chilled.
Serving: 1 glass

Nutritional Value: Anti-inflammatory, high in vitamin C, and aids digestion.
Preparation Time: 5 minutes

25. Beetroot-Carrot-Apple Refresher

Ingredients:
- 1 beetroot
- 2 carrots
- 1 green apple
- 1 tablespoon lemon juice

Instructions:
1. Wash and peel the beetroot, carrots, and green apple.
2. Cut them into smaller pieces.
3. Add the beetroot, carrots, green apple, and lemon juice to your juicer.
4. Stir well and serve over ice.

Serving: 1 glass
Nutritional Value: High in antioxidants, vitamins A and C, and supports liver health.
Preparation Time: 5 minutes

26. Blueberry-Avocado Delight

Ingredients:
- 1 cup blueberries
- 1 ripe avocado
- 1 cup almond milk
- 1 tablespoon honey (optional)

Instructions:
1. Wash the blueberries.
2. Cut the avocado in half, remove the pit, and scoop out the flesh.
3. Add the blueberries, avocado, almond milk, and honey (if desired) to a blender.
4. Blend until smooth.
5. Serve chilled.

Serving: 1 glass
Nutritional Value: High in antioxidants, quality fats, and fiber.
Preparation Time: 5 minutes

27. Lemon-Ginger Cleanser

Ingredients:
- 3 lemons (juiced)
- 1-inch piece of ginger
- 1 tablespoon honey (optional)

- Pinch of cayenne pepper (optional)
Instructions:
1. Juice the lemons.
2. Peel and slice the ginger.
3. Add the lemon juice, ginger, honey (if desired), and cayenne pepper (if desired) to your juicer.
4. Stir well and serve chilled.
Serving: 1 glass
Nutritional Value: Detoxifying, aids digestion, and boosts immune function.
Preparation Time: 5 minutes

28. Pomegranate-Kale Powerhouse

Ingredients:
- 1 cup pomegranate seeds
- 2 cups kale leaves
- 1 green apple
- 1 tablespoon lime juice
Instructions:
1. Wash the pomegranate seeds and kale leaves.
2. Cut the green apple into smaller pieces.

3. Add the pomegranate seeds, kale leaves, green apple, and lime juice to your juicer.

4. Stir well and serve over ice.

Serving: 1 glass

Nutritional Value: High in antioxidants, vitamins A and C, and aids digestion.

Preparation Time: 5 minutes

29. Pear-Cucumber-Mint Cooler

Ingredients:

- 2 pears
- 1 cucumber
- 1 handful of fresh mint leaves
- 1 tablespoon lime juice

Instructions:

1. Wash the pears, cucumber, and mint leaves.

2. Cut the pears and cucumber into smaller pieces.

3. Add the pears, cucumber, mint leaves, and lime juice to your juicer.

4. Stir well and serve over ice.

Serving: 1 glass

Nutritional Value: Refreshing, hydrating, and rich in vitamins and minerals.

Preparation Time: 5 minutes

30. Ginger-Turmeric-Apple Elixir

Ingredients:
- 1-inch piece of ginger
- 1-inch piece of turmeric root
- 2 green apples
- 1 lemon (juiced)

Instructions:
1. Wash the ginger, turmeric root, and apples.
2. Slice the ginger and turmeric root.
3. Cut the apples into smaller pieces.
4. Add the ginger, turmeric root, apples, and lemon juice to your juicer.
5. Stir well and serve chilled.

Serving: 1 glass

Nutritional Value: Anti-inflammatory, aids digestion, and boosts immune function.

Preparation Time: 5 minutes

Chapter 2: 30 mouthwatering Smoothie Recipes for asthma

1. Strawberry Banana Blast

Ingredients:
- 1 cup strawberries
- 1 ripe banana
- 1 cup almond milk
- 1 tablespoon honey (optional)

Instructions:
1. Blend all the ingredients together until smooth.
2. Serve immediately.

Serving: 1 smoothie
Nutritional Value: Calories: 180, Carbohydrates: 43g, Protein: 2g, Fat: 2g
Cooking Time: 5 minutes

2. Mango Ginger Zing

Ingredients:
- 1 ripe mango
- 1-inch piece of fresh ginger

- 1 cup coconut water
- ½ cup plain Greek yogurt
Instructions:
1. Peel and chop the mango.
2. Grate the ginger.
3. Combine all the ingredients in a blender and blend until smooth.
4. Serve chilled.
Serving: 1 smoothie
Nutritional Value: Calories: 230, Carbohydrates: 45g, Protein: 12g, Fat: 2g
Cooking Time: 5 minutes

3. Green Powerhouse

Ingredients:
- 1 cup spinach
- 1 ripe pear
- ½ cucumber
- 1 cup almond milk
- 1 tablespoon chia seeds
Instructions:
1. Wash the spinach leaves.
2. Peel and chop the pear.
3. Peel and slice the cucumber.

4. Blend all the combinations of the ingredients until well combined.

5. Add more almond milk if needed to adjust the consistency.

Serving: 1 smoothie

Nutritional Value: Calories: 180, Carbohydrates: 35g, Protein: 5g, Fat: 4g

Cooking Time: 5 minutes

4. Pineapple Mint Refresher

Ingredients:
- 1 cup pineapple chunks
- ½ cup fresh mint leaves
- 1 cup coconut water
- Juice of 1 lime

Instructions:

1. Blend all the ingredients together until smooth.

2. Serve over ice for a refreshing twist.

Serving: 1 smoothie

Nutritional Value: Calories: 140, Carbohydrates: 35g, Protein: 2g, Fat: 1g

Cooking Time: 5 minutes

5. Blueberry Avocado Dream

Ingredients:
- 1 cup blueberries
- 1 ripe avocado
- 1 cup almond milk
- 1 tablespoon honey (optional)

Instructions:
1. Blend all the ingredients together until smooth.
2. Add more almond milk if needed to adjust the consistency.
3. Serve chilled.

Serving: 1 smoothie

Nutritional Value: Calories: 280, Carbohydrates: 30g, Protein: 6g, Fat: 17g

Cooking Time: 5 minutes

6. Carrot Orange Delight

Ingredients:
- 2 carrots
- 2 oranges (peeled and deseeded)
- ½ cup coconut water
- 1 tablespoon flax seeds

Instructions:
1. Peel and chop the carrots.
2. Juice the oranges.
3. Combine all the ingredients together and blend till smooth.
4. Serve chilled.
Serving: 1 smoothie
Nutritional Value: Calories: 150, Carbohydrates: 34g, Protein: 3g, Fat: 1g
Cooking Time: 5 minutes

7. Kiwi Berry Blast

Ingredients:
- 2 kiwis (peeled and sliced)
- 1 cup of different berries (strawberries, raspberries, and blueberries)
- 1 cup almond milk
- 1 tablespoon honey (optional)
Instructions:
1. Blend all the ingredients together until smooth.
2. Serve over ice for a cool treat.
Serving: 1 smoothie
Nutritional Value: Calories: 160, Carbohydrates: 38g, Protein: 3g, Fat: 1g

Cooking Time: 5 minutes

8. Spinach Pineapple Paradise

Ingredients:
- 1 cup spinach
- 1 cup pineapple chunks
- 1 ripe banana
- 1 cup coconut water

Instructions:
1. Wash the spinach leaves.
2. Blend all the ingredients together until smooth.
3. Add more coconut water if needed to adjust the consistency.

Serving: 1 smoothie

Nutritional Value: Calories: 210, Carbohydrates: 52g, Protein: 3g, Fat: 1g

Cooking Time: 5 minutes

9. Raspberry Almond Delight

Ingredients:
- 1 cup raspberries
- 1 cup almond milk
- ¼ cup almonds

- 1 tablespoon honey (optional)

Instructions:

1. Blend all the ingredients together until smooth.

2. Serve chilled.

Serving: 1 smoothie

Nutritional Value: Calories: 200, Carbohydrates: 28g, Protein: 5g, Fat: 8g

Cooking Time: 5 minutes

10. Turmeric Mango Magic

Ingredients:

- 1 cup mango chunks
- 1 cup coconut milk
- 1 teaspoon turmeric powder
- 1 teaspoon honey (optional)

Instructions:

1. Blend all the ingredients together until smooth.

2. Serve chilled.

Serving: 1 smoothie

Nutritional Value: Calories: 220, Carbohydrates: 35g, Protein: 1g, Fat: 10g

Cooking Time: 5 minutes

11. Cherry Vanilla Bliss

Ingredients:
- 1 cup cherries (pitted)
- 1 cup almond milk
- ½ teaspoon vanilla extract
- 1 tablespoon honey (optional)

Instructions:
1. Blend all the ingredients together until smooth.
2. Serve chilled.

Serving: 1 smoothie

Nutritional Value: Calories: 160, Carbohydrates: 36g, Protein: 2g, Fat: 3g

Cooking Time: 5 minutes

12. Beet Berry Boost

Ingredients:
- 1 small cooked beet
- 1 cup of different berries (strawberries, and blueberries)
- 1 cup almond milk
- 1 tablespoon honey (optional)

Instructions:

1. Blend all the ingredients together until smooth.

2. Serve chilled.

Serving: 1 smoothie

Nutritional Value: Calories: 200, Carbohydrates: 45g, Protein: 3g, Fat: 2g

Cooking Time: 5 minutes

13. Papaya Coconut Splash

Ingredients:

- 1 cup papaya chunks
- ½ cup coconut milk
- 1 tablespoon lime juice
- 1 tablespoon shredded coconut

Instructions:

1. Blend all the ingredients together until smooth.

2. Serve chilled and garnish with shredded coconut.

Serving: 1 smoothie

Nutritional Value: Calories: 190, Carbohydrates: 35g, Protein: 2g, Fat: 7g

Cooking Time: 5 minutes

14. Peach Oatmeal Delight

Ingredients:
- 1 ripe peach
- ½ cup rolled oats
- 1 cup almond milk
- 1 tablespoon honey (optional)

Instructions:
1. Peel and chop the peach.
2. Combine all the ingredients and blend until smooth and well combined.
3. Serve chilled.

Serving: 1 smoothie

Nutritional Value: Calories: 260, Carbohydrates: 50g, Protein: 7g, Fat: 4g

Cooking Time: 5 minutes

14. Peach Oatmeal Delight

Ingredients:
- 2 oranges (peeled and deseeded)
- 2 carrots
- 1 cup coconut water
- 1 tablespoon chia seeds

Instructions:
1. Juice the oranges.

2. Peel and chop the carrots.

3. Blend all the ingredients together until smooth.

4. Serve chilled.

Serving: 1 smoothie

Nutritional Value: Calories: 180, Carbohydrates: 40g, Protein: 5g, Fat: 2g

Cooking Time: 5 minutes

16. Kale Berry Blast

Ingredients:
- 1 cup kale leaves
- 1 cup of different berries (strawberries, raspberries, and blueberries)
- 1 cup almond milk
- 1 tablespoon honey (optional)

Instructions:

1. Wash the kale leaves.

2. Juice all the ingredients together until well combined.

3. Add more almond milk if needed to adjust the consistency.

Serving: 1 smoothie

Nutritional Value: Calories: 180, Carbohydrates: 38g, Protein: 4g, Fat: 2g

Cooking Time: 5 minutes

17. Watermelon Mint Cooler

Ingredients:
- 2 cups watermelon chunks
- ½ cup fresh mint leaves
- Juice of 1 lime
- 1 tablespoon honey (optional)

Instructions:
1. Blend all the ingredients together until smooth.
2. Serve over ice for a refreshing treat.

Serving: 1 smoothie
Nutritional Value: Calories: 120, Carbohydrates: 31g, Protein: 2g, Fat: 1g
Cooking Time: 5 minutes

18. Apple Cinnamon Delight

Ingredients:
- 1 apple, cored and chopped
- 1 ripe banana
- 1/2 cup of almond milk (or any other non-dairy milk of your choice)
- A handful of spinach

- 1 teaspoon of cinnamon
- A drizzle of honey (optional, adjust to taste)
- Ice cubes

Instructions

1. In a blender, combine 1 apple (cored and chopped), 1 ripe banana, 1/2 cup of almond milk, a handful of spinach, 1 teaspoon of cinnamon, and a drizzle of honey.
2. Add a few ice cubes to chill the smoothie.
3. Blend until smooth and creamy.
4. Pour into a glass and sprinkle a pinch of cinnamon on top for extra aroma and flavor.

Serving: 1 smoothie

Nutritional Value: Calories: 120, Carbohydrates: 31g, Protein: 2g, Fat: 1g

Cooking Time: 15 minutes

19. Mango Coconut Smoothie

Ingredients:

- 1 cup frozen mango chunks
- 1/2 cup coconut milk

- 1/2 cup Greek yogurt
- 1 tablespoon honey
- 1/4 teaspoon turmeric (optional)
Instructions:
1. Combine all the ingredients in a blender.
2. Blend until smooth and creamy.
3. Pour into a glass and serve.
Serving size: 1 smoothie
Nutritional value: Calories: 270, Carbohydrates: 43g, Protein: 11g, Fat: 7g
Preparation time: 5 minutes

20. Spinach Banana Smoothie

Ingredients:
- 1 ripe banana
- 1 cup spinach
- 1/2 cup almond milk
- 1 tablespoon almond butter
- 1 tablespoon honey
Instructions:
1. Put all ingredients in a blender.
2. Blend until well combined and smooth.
3. Pour into a glass and enjoy.

Serving size: 1 smoothie
Nutritional value: Calories: 230, Carbohydrates: 45g, Protein: 4g, Fat: 5g
Preparation time: 5 minutes

21. Raspberry Almond Smoothie

Ingredients:
- 1 cup frozen raspberries
- 1/2 cup almond milk
- 1/2 cup Greek yogurt
- 1 tablespoon almond butter
- 1 tablespoon honey

Instructions:
1. Put all the ingredients in a blender.
2. Blend until creamy and smooth.
3. Pour into a glass and serve.

Serving size: 1 smoothie
Nutritional value: Calories: 280, Carbohydrates: 39g, Protein: 12g, Fat: 10g
Preparation time: 5 minutes

22. Kiwi Lime Smoothie

Ingredients:
- 2 kiwis, peeled
- Juice of 1 lime
- 1 ripe banana
- 1 cup coconut water
- 1 tablespoon honey

Instructions:
1. Combine all the ingredients in a blender.
2. Blend until well combined and smooth.
3. Pour into a glass and enjoy.

Serving size: 1 smoothie

Nutritional value: Calories: 200, Carbohydrates: 48g, Protein: 2g, Fat: 1g

Preparation time: 5 minutes

23. Peach Oatmeal Smoothie

Ingredients:
- 1 ripe peach, pitted and sliced
- 1/2 cup rolled oats
- 1 cup almond milk
- 1 tablespoon honey

- 1/4 teaspoon cinnamon
Instructions
1. Combine all the ingredients inside a blender.
2. Blend until smooth and creamy.
3. Pour into a glass and enjoy.
Serving size: 1 smoothie
Nutritional value: Calories: 260, Carbohydrates: 52g, Protein: 6g, Fat: 4g
Preparation time: 7 minutes

24. Carrot Ginger Smoothie

Ingredients
- 1 carrot, peeled and chopped
- 1 inch fresh ginger, peeled
- 1 orange, peeled
- 1/2 cup coconut water
- 1 tablespoon honey
Instructions
1. Combine all the ingredients in a blender.
2. Blend until well combined and smooth.
3. Pour into a glass and serve.
Serving size: 1 smoothie

Nutritional value: Calories: 160, Carbohydrates: 38g, Protein: 2g, Fat: 0g
Preparation time: 5 minutes

25. Apple Cinnamon Smoothie

Ingredients:
- 1 apple, cored and diced
- 1/2 cup Greek yogurt
- 1 cup almond milk
- 1 tablespoon honey
- 1/4 teaspoon cinnamon

Instructions:
1. Put together all the ingredients in a blender.
2. Blend till creamy and we'll combined.
3. Pour into a glass and enjoy.
Serving size: 1 smoothie
Nutritional value: Calories: 210, Carbohydrates: 44g, Protein: 8g, Fat: 2g
Preparation time: 5 minutes

26. Spinach Mango Smoothie

Ingredients:
- 1 cup spinach

- 1 cup frozen mango chunks
- 1/2 cup coconut water
- 1 tablespoon chia seeds
- 1 tablespoon honey

Instructions:

1. Unite all the ingredients in a blender.

2. Blend until well combined and creamy.

3. Pour into a glass and serve.

Serving size: 1 smoothie

Nutritional value: Calories: 220, Carbohydrates: 48g, Protein: 4g, Fat: 3g

Preparation time: 5 minutes

27. Peanut Butter Banana Smoothie

Ingredients:

- 1 ripe banana
- 2 tablespoons peanut butter
- 1 cup almond milk
- 1 tablespoon honey
- 1/4 teaspoon vanilla extract

Instructions:

1. Put together all the ingredients in a blender.

2. Blend until well combined and smooth.

3. Pour into a glass and enjoy.

Serving size: 1 smoothie

Nutritional value: Calories: 360, Carbohydrates: 40g, Protein: 10g, Fat: 20g

Preparation time: 5 minutes

28. Watermelon Mint Smoothie

Ingredients:
- 2 cups diced watermelon
- 1 tablespoon fresh mint leaves
- 1/2 cup coconut water
- 1 tablespoon lime juice
- 1 tablespoon honey

Instructions:

1. Combine all the ingredients in a blender.

2. Blend until smooth and well combined.

3. Pour into a glass and serve.

Serving size: 1 smoothie

Nutritional value: Calories: 120, Carbohydrates: 30g, Protein: 2g, Fat: 0g

Preparation time: 5 minutes

29. Cherry Vanilla Smoothie

Ingredients:
- 1 cup frozen cherries
- 1/2 cup Greek yogurt
- 1 cup almond milk
- 1 tablespoon honey
- 1/2 teaspoon vanilla extract

Instructions:
1. Unite all the ingredients in a blender.
2. Blend until creamy and well mixed.
3. Pour into a glass and enjoy.

Serving size: 1 smoothie
Nutritional value: Calories: 220, Carbohydrates: 39g, Protein: 10g, Fat: 4g
Preparation time: 5 minutes

30. Blueberry Kale Smoothie

Ingredients:
- 1 cup blueberries
- 1 cup chopped kale
- 1/2 cup almond milk

- 1 tablespoon almond butter
- 1 tablespoon honey
Instructions:
1. Put together all the ingredients in a blender.
2. Blend until well combined and smooth.
3. Pour into a glass and serve.
Serving size: 1 smoothie
Nutritional value: Calories: 230, Carbohydrates: 43g, Protein: 5g, Fat: 5g
Preparation time: 5 minutes

Chapter 3: Bonus

21 must know precautions for an asthmatic patient

Here are 21 general precautions that may be beneficial for asthma patients:

1. Regular Medical Check-ups: Schedule regular check-ups with your healthcare provider to monitor and manage your asthma effectively.

2. Understand Triggers: Identify and understand your asthma triggers, such as allergens, pollutants, or specific activities, and take steps to avoid them.

3. Create an Asthma Action Plan: Work with your healthcare provider to develop a personalized asthma action plan that outlines steps to take during both routine and exacerbation periods.

4. Stay Informed: Keep yourself informed about the latest advancements in asthma treatment and management.

5. Medication Compliance: Take your prescribed medications as directed, and inform your healthcare provider if you experience any side effects.

6. Allergy Management: Manage allergies effectively, as they can exacerbate asthma symptoms. Undergo allergy testing to identify specific triggers.

7. Regular Exercise: Engage in regular, moderate exercise as approved by your healthcare provider to improve lung function and overall health.

8. Proper Warm-up and Cool-down: Always warm up before exercising and cool down afterward to minimize the risk of asthma symptoms during physical activity.

9. Adequate Hydration: Stay well-hydrated to maintain optimal respiratory function.

10. Inhaler Technique: Learn and practice proper inhaler techniques to ensure effective medication delivery.

11. Avoid Smoking and Secondhand Smoke: Avoid smoking, and steer clear of environments with secondhand smoke, as it can worsen asthma symptoms.

12. Clean Indoor Air: Ensure good indoor air quality by minimizing exposure to pollutants, using air purifiers, and ventilating living spaces.

13. Healthy Diet: Maintain a well-balanced diet rich in fruits, vegetables, and omega-3 fatty acids, which may have anti-inflammatory properties.

14. Stress Management: Practice stress-reducing techniques such as meditation, yoga, or deep breathing exercises.

15. Weather Awareness: Be mindful of weather conditions, especially extreme temperatures and high humidity, which can impact asthma symptoms.

16. Flu Vaccination: Get an annual flu vaccination to reduce the risk of respiratory infections that can trigger asthma attacks.

17. Bedding and Pillow Covers: Use allergen-proof bedding and pillow covers to minimize exposure to dust mites.

18. Emergency Preparedness: Have an emergency kit with your rescue inhaler, medication list, and contact information for your healthcare provider readily accessible.

19. Avoid Strong Odors and Irritants: Steer clear of strong odors, perfumes, and other irritants that may trigger asthma symptoms.

20. Monitor Peak Flow: Regularly monitor your peak flow to track changes in lung function and adjust your management plan accordingly.

21. Educate Others: Ensure that family, friends, and colleagues are aware of your condition and know how to respond in case of an asthma emergency.

Note

This list is a general guide, and individuals with asthma should consult with their healthcare providers for personalized advice based on their specific health needs and circumstances.

Conclusion

As we wrap up "Asthma Juicing and Smoothies for Beginners," remember: each sip is a step towards breathing easier and living a fuller life. This book isn't just a guide; it's a roadmap to respiratory vitality. Carry with you the knowledge that these recipes are more than blends – they're your allies in the journey to a healthier, more vibrant you. Cheers to your path to better breathing, one sip at a time!